EMMA ROSE SPARROW

Autumn's Display

By Emma Rose Sparrow

Publish Date: November 9, 2015

Editor-in-Chief: Connor Chagnon
Sterling Elle Publishing
Bradford, Massachusetts

ISBN-13:978-1519216564
ISBN-10:1519216564

AUTUMN'S DISPLAY

An Emma Rose Sparrow Book

AUTUMN'S DISPLAY follows the events of a woman on a gorgeous autumn morning. With a wonderful destination and a plan to fill the day with fun, she sets out.

Join her in all of the delights of autumn; and you, like her, may come across a few surprises as well.

If you are an adult bookworm who is looking for an interesting read or a book lover that enjoys a book that can be read over and over, this book is for you.

It is hoped that you find this book worthy of adding to your collection.

Enjoy your read!

TABLE OF CONTENTS

ACKNOWLEDGMENTS

Don't you just love the fact that a good book can instantly bring you somewhere new? And this happens without the stress and strain of actual travel.

Books allow us to visit other places for a while and then be right back in our comfortable chairs whenever we wish.

For thousands of years, writers have worked to bring the joy of reading to those who appreciate a good story. Each year, hundreds of authors take their first try at writing and thousands of bookworms bring those books into their homes.

Great gratitude is given to all of the authors in the world. And a huge "thank you" is given to all of the book lovers around the globe.

If it were not for readers like you, the art of writing would be lost.

~Emma Rose Sparrow

CHAPTER 1: PETUNIAS, NOT POTATOES

I tried to not let the disappointment show in my voice. "No, no, it's okay," I reassured my neighbor through the phone, "Obviously you need to see the hair stylist today. And my gosh, please don't ever again fall asleep with your hair plastered in lemon juice. What were you thinking?"

She explained her theory that the lemon was supposed to stay on for 10 minutes. It was to give her 'youthful blond highlights'. And falling asleep wasn't part of the plan.

She went on a little bit longer, expressing her biggest worry. "No," I answered, "I don't think they'll have to go to such extremes as to shave it all off."

After wishing her luck, I plopped down on the sofa. I rubbed my eyes and took in a deep breath. That was exhausting! She was my fifth phone call of the morning.

The phone was not being my friend today. In fact, it was downright against me.

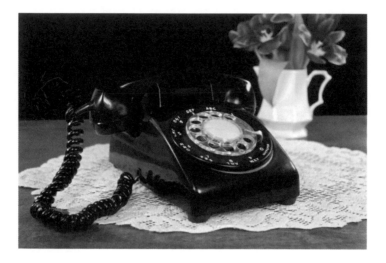

I had tried my friend Clara, head of the gardening committee. "Potatoes! Do you believe it?", she spat out, quite flustered, "They dumped over 1000 potatoes out on the drive instead of delivering a box of 100 petunia seed packages to the door! I'm up to my eyeballs in spuds. This will take me forever to sort out."

I tried my daughter. "Well, I've only three more hours of baking and perhaps two more hours of icing after that. Ah-choo! The sprinkles and such may take another hour at the most. Ah-choo! I can try to hurry that, though. A... A.... Ah-choo!" Almond flour had drifted up into her nose.

I had tried my friend Elizabeth. "If you wouldn't be so stubborn about trying out Bingo Meets Pokeno, you could join us today!" she exclaimed. "And I've been thinking about how I can incorporate knitting and checkers. Maybe you'll like that better?"

So, as you can see, neither the phone nor the circumstances of those that I reached out to were being corporative.

I was on my own today. So, what would I do?

The answer, in part, came from looking out of the large bay window.

EMMA ROSE SPARROW

CHAPTER 2: TIME TO REDISCOVER

The bay window of my living room offered me a wonderful view of the wooded park across the street. Autumn's foliage was in full force. The display of color was amazing.

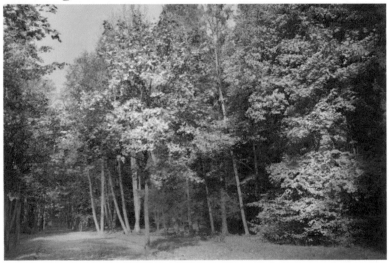

The park contained a nice paved walking path. In addition, near the center would be a small, pretty body of water. The path would bring me around in a big loop encircling the small forested land. And if I so chose, access into the deeper part of the forest was rather easy as well. Soft grass without many obstacles would allow me to walk inward, should I wish to.

It had been cloudy with sprinkles the last four days in a row. But now, on this wonderful autumn morning, the sun shone bright.

I could see that the light rain had dislodged lots of dazzling leaves from the trees. And that would afford me more of a chance to win the game.

"What game?" you may ask. Well, forever since I can remember, from when I was a young child, I played a certain autumn game. And when I had met my husband and we took romantic walks on crisp fall weekends, I'd played it with him.

As the years tumbled by and I was blessed

with my children, I'd bring them out to the playground after school on refreshing autumn days. We'd stomp through the thick blanket of leaves on the ground. We'd make piles to jump in. We'd throw heaps of leaves at each other, laughing as we did. But we always kept the game in mind.

As time slipped by, faster and faster, as it does for most of us, I had let the game slip by as well. It was a long forgotten piece of 'something I used to do'. I hadn't thought about it for years. 'Why was that?' I asked myself.

Autumn is one of the loveliest seasons and it was time that I rediscovered the simple joys it could bring.

EMMA ROSE SPARROW

CHAPTER 3: COLOR FROM ALL SIDES

It didn't take me long to get ready. Once I had reminded myself of how lovely it would be to take a walk and play my autumn game, I was quick on my feet.

'What game?' you may still be asking. Well, it's rather simplistic in nature. Don't make fun of me here, okay? The rules are easy. The first part is to find a perfect fallen leaf of each of the following colors: Red, yellow, orange and tan. While tan may seem a tad boring, it was after all, a part of autumn.

The second part of this is a bit trickier. For each leaf that I find, I will then need to find a matching object. This can be a person, animal or any other thing whose colors match the 'perfect' leaf.

As I crossed the street to meet up with the walking path, I took a moment to take in the sight before me. The woodland looked enchanting. It was as if a painter had set up an enormous canvas. And I had the pleasure of watching him as he moved the brush.

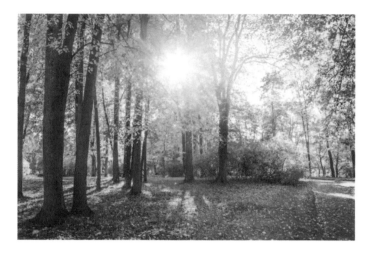

As the sun's ray bounced between the tall branches, I imagined his paint brush adjusting. As leaves drifted downward in gentle, waving arcs, I envisioned that the artist was dabbing the canvas.

Now, I would be part of the picture myself. I was looking forward to what I would be able to spy.

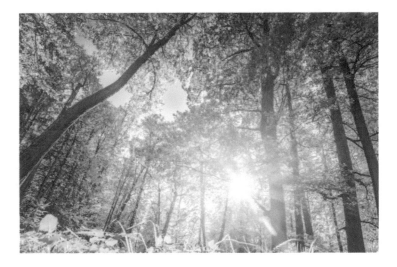

    With colors surrounding me from all sides and from above, there was no shortage of possibilities.

CHAPTER 4: CRIMSON RED

Just as I wondered which color would call out to me first, I glanced to the side and received my answer. A Maple tree. Its branches were extending out over the pathway. They were like arms, reaching across to show off its attire.

Each leaf popped with a shiny, glistening red.

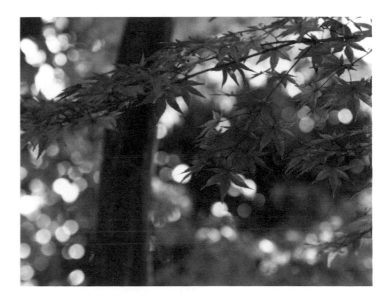

And my search of the ground to find a pretty red leaf was underway.

In no rush and planning on taking my time, I scanned the soft, earthy carpet of the woods.

And there it was.

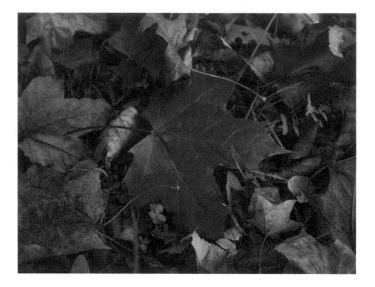

Amidst crumbled, dried leaves that may have once held a regal color, a soft red leaf lay proudly on top. Perfect!

And on it went. Within 20 minutes or so, I had gathered my red, yellow, orange and tan leaves.

Now that I had my small collection, the next order of business was to find matching objects.

The park was quite popular with people of all ages. It was a pleasant place to have a picnic near the water. And a nice, safe place to stretch one's legs. The bounty of trees provided lots of areas for wildlife. So while I was not sure of what I would find, I was confident that I would match some, if not all, of my leaves.

A flutter got my attention and I knew to stay still. If a pretty bird had landed near me, I'd be wise to not scare it off until I was able to determine its color.

I knew better than to expect to see a robin. Though it would have matched the red leaf that I had found, a robin sighting in autumn would be rare. While some robins ventured north to find berries as winter approached, in my area they were strictly a springtime bird.

I slowly looked over. First with one eye and then with both. It was even better than a robin!

To my pleasant surprise, I saw that it was a Scarlet Tanager.

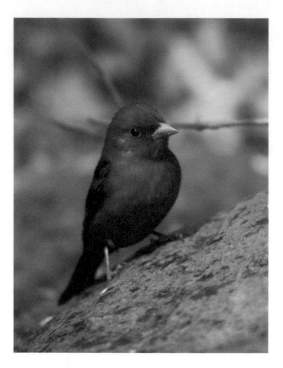

Now, let me tell you why this was such a surprise! There are 3 reasons:

First, this was a male Scarlet Tanager, the most colorful of the two genders. However, this is not always so. As fall tumbles into winter, he loses his red plumage. The red slowly turns to a yellow-green, which then matches what the females look like. But this bird still held his bright crimson-red feathers.

In just another month or so, it would be a different story.

The second reason why it was a treat to spy this amazing red bird was due to his normal behavior. Scarlet Tanager birds tend to stay very high up in the trees. Typically, they perch in the treetops, only to soar out to capture insects flying by. Only rarely do they visit the forest floor. Yet, here he was.

The third and final reason why this sighting was so special is because come October, the Scarlet Tanager makes its way south. Some go as far south as South America. In another week or two, he would be gone.

So, seeing this beautiful red bird that matched my red leaf was indeed a treat!

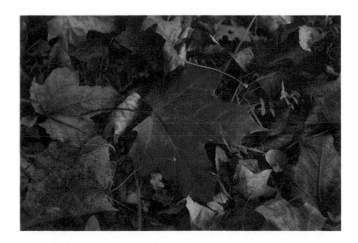

CHAPTER 5: YELLOW BONUS

Enjoying my stroll through the wonderland that is autumn, I clutched the leaves that I had gathered. With such vivid colors all around me, the trick was to spot a certain color other than the amazing leaves.

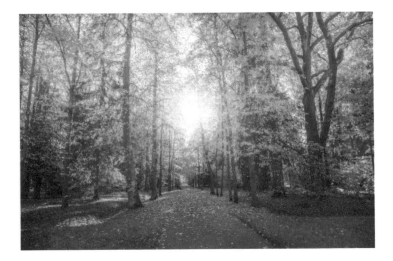

I was pleased with my progress so far. I had spotted the red Scarlet Tanager bird that matched my red leaf. What would be next?

Plodding down the sidewalk a few more steps, a sweet, giggling voice got my attention.

However, I couldn't have missed the next sight even with my eyes closed.

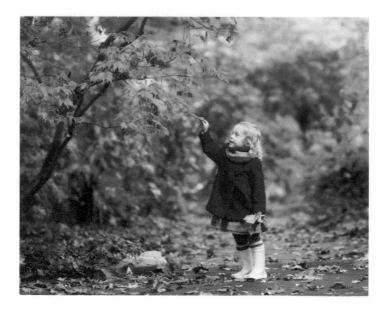

A beautiful little girl with a bright red coat and bright yellow boots! Yellow boots, that would do! They would match the yellow leaf I had found. And even if she didn't have a splotch of yellow on her, I still would have stopped.

This precious little girl was collecting leaves just as I was. "Look!" she yelled out to me, "The trees are shedding! Come look!"

I smiled as I approached. Glancing to the side, I spotted her mother, who was tending to a second, younger child. She gave me a quick, friendly nod as if to say, "It's fine!"

"Shedding?" I inquired, as I stepped closer, "Like a puppy?"

"Oh, yes," she replied, quite serious, "They are shedding to get ready for snowfall time!"

"That they are," I agreed.

She showed me the leaves that she had found so far. When she asked to see the leaves that I held, she let out a gasp. "One of every color! That's what I'll do too!"

"Wait," she continued on, "If the trees are shedding, which they are... Won't they be cold in snowfall time?" She suddenly looked worried.

"That's a good question," I replied, "But,

unlike a puppy, these trees are not just shedding, they are getting ready to go to sleep. They'll sleep right through the snow. And when they wake in the springtime, they won't even know what happened!"

She seemed pleased with my answer. But then she innocently asked, "Sleep right through? Like when daddy says he sleeps through Gram-gram's visits and doesn't miss anything at all?"

I suppressed a giggle, looking over to her mother. The woman gave me a 'What are you gonna do?' look and I responded to the mother with a smile and a shrug. "Something like that," I replied to the child.

Though I could have stayed all day, it was time to get going. I thanked the young girl for allowing me to visit with her.

As I turned to leave, she scrambled up a small hill with the energy that only the youth can have.

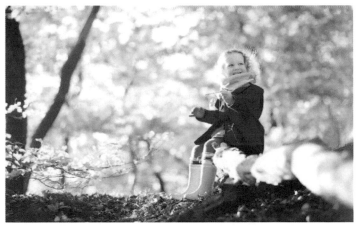

I waved an enthusiastic 'good bye', hoping I'd run into her another day. Having her yellow boots match the yellow leaf I'd found was a bonus. That little girl was a darling!

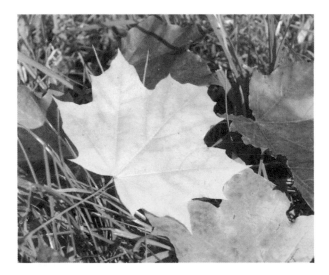

CHAPTER 6: FAIRYDIDDLES

So far the day was a success. Walking through the park on the most beautiful of fall days, I had found a leaf of each color. Red, yellow, orange and tan. I'd bring them home once my game was done. Perhaps I'd press them in a book.

In my quest to locate things that matched my chosen leaves, at this point my goal was half complete. I had seen a gorgeous red Scarlet Tanager bird. And I had the pleasure of meeting a cute little girl with bright yellow boots.

As I rounded the corner, I slowed my pace just a bit. If I finished looping around the park too quickly, I wouldn't have a chance to find matching objects for orange and tan.

Orange would be a tricky one. There were

very few things in the environment that were naturally orange. Most likely, I would need to spy something manmade.

I saw something and it grabbed my attention. Did it match one of my leaves? No, not at all. It was a bench and boy did I need to rest my tootsies.

As I sat down to take a little break, I drew in a slow breath of crisp autumn air. It was both invigorating and relaxing at the same time. I found myself lost in thought, as I took in the scenery around me.

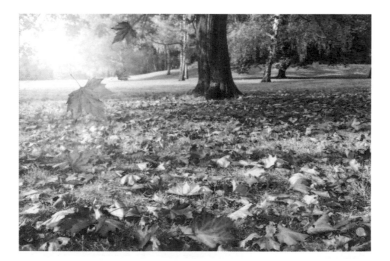

Isn't it funny how if you were smack in the middle of summer and suddenly you felt the cool winds of the fall, you'd believe it to be frigid? Yet, when you are gently guided to it, day by day, little by little, it feels wonderful.

Another thought that I had, I admit, was not my own original thought. It was something that my daughter had told me once. Many others have supposed the same. And perhaps you have thought this yourself.

She had said, "Mom, I think I know why the trees turn to such beautiful colors in the fall. It's because nature wants to give us something splendid… a sort of present, if you will. To make us happy before things have to be cold and bleak for the winter."

And with that, I could not argue. And I'm quite sure that you will not as well.

I was about to glance down at the leaves I had collected when I spotted movement from the corner of my eye.

Perfect!

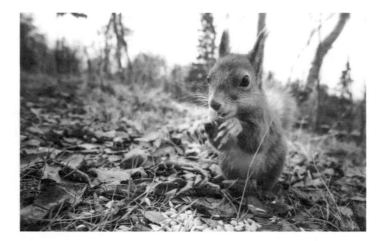

Right there before me, was a North American Red Squirrel. Now, never mind his name, because his orange fur was just the thing that I had wanted to find.

These cute little guys have several funny nicknames. Among their nicknames are 'boomers' and 'chickarees'. If that's not amusing enough, another nickname for these woodland marvels are 'fairydiddles'. I think that I like fairydiddles the most.

Glancing down at my autumn leaf collection, I confirmed that he matched my orange leaf just fine.

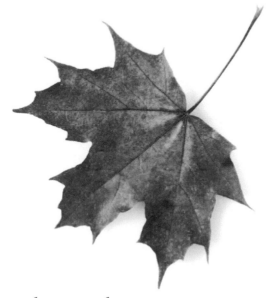

Three down and one to go.

CHAPTER 7: LAUGHS & LICKS

As I walked along the path, the small pond sat to my left. Once again, I took care to slow my pace, in an effort to extend this outing as long as possible.

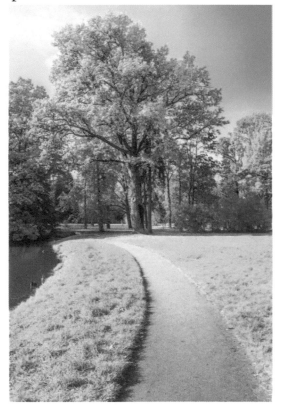

At the large tree up ahead, I would veer right and within just a few minutes, be back home. I still had the tan leaf to match up to something. My mind started running through things that are tan.

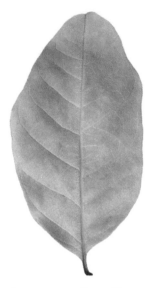

Well, sand... and dirt. Twigs and branches. None of those were particularly interesting. Yet, if I reached the end of the path without better options, I would choose one of those to match my tan leaf. I hated to leave things undone. No pun intended.

With that thought, I suddenly got the sense that someone was watching me. Does that ever happen to you? I casually scanned the area. There were a few people scattered about, however none seemed to be looking my way.

And that's when I realized, I was scanning too high. There, at ground level, was the cutest Beagle puppy I had ever seen. Just resting there, looking at me, with sweet innocent eyes.

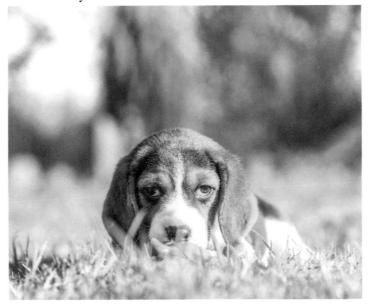

His coat was a shiny blend of 'hound dog' colors. Surely the tans would count as matching my tan leaf! And it couldn't have come in a sweeter package.

He was very shy, and stayed planted right where he was as I gently approached to pet him. With a soft breath, he nudged his nose into the palm of my hand. This little puppy was soaking up every moment of attention.

I stayed beside him for much longer than my growling stomach had wanted. And it was only when his owners had come over to bring him back to their car, that I decided it was time for me to go as well. Lunch was waiting!

What a pleasant venture this had been. I had collected leaves of every color. I spotted a red Scarlet Tanager bird. Yellow came in the way of a lovely young girl with bright yellow boots.

I found orange in the fur of a cute little squirrel. And the puppy with tan in his soft coat rounded things out.

There was only one more thing to do.

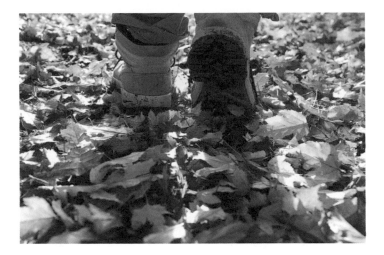

I enthusiastically crunched the fallen leaves all the way back home. After all, walking over a carpet of crispy, colorful leaves was yet another joy of autumn.

ABOUT THE AUTHOR

Emma Rose Sparrow lives in a small New England coastal town with her two sons. She enjoys many creative ventures, including design and writing. She wishes to personally thank each and every one of her book readers for keeping the art of reading alive.

OTHER BOOKS IN THIS SERIES BY EMMA ROSE SPARROW

What the Wind Showed to Me

The Sandy Shoreline

A Dusting of Snow

Three Things

Down by the Meadow

Made in the USA
Lexington, KY
15 June 2017